Active at Any Age:

A Beginner's Guide to Overcoming a Sedentary Lifestyle

By

Rosanna C. Hernandez

TABLE OF CONTENTS

Introduction

Welcome to "Active at Any Age: A Beginner's Guide to Overcoming a Sedentary Lifestyle." This book is your gateway to a healthier, more vibrant life, no matter your age or current fitness level. Whether you're just starting to think about incorporating physical activity into your routine or looking to rekindle your commitment to staying active, you've taken an important first step by picking up this guide.

The Sedentary Epidemic

In our modern world, many of us spend long hours sitting—whether at a desk, in front of a screen, or commuting. This sedentary lifestyle can lead to a host of health issues, including weight gain, cardiovascular disease, diabetes, and even mental health challenges like anxiety and depression. But the good news is that it's never too late to make a change.

The Power of Movement

Physical activity is one of the most effective ways to combat the negative effects of a sedentary lifestyle. It improves not only physical health by reducing the risk of chronic diseases and enhancing muscle strength, bone density, and joint health, but also boosts mental well-being by reducing stress, improving mood, and increasing energy levels. Movement is a powerful tool that can significantly enhance the quality of your life.

This Book Is for You

Whether you're a complete beginner or someone who's fallen out of the habit of regular exercise, this book is designed to provide you with practical, actionable advice. We'll explore the science behind the benefits of physical activity, offer tips for getting started, and address common barriers to staying active. You'll find guidance on creating a personalized exercise routine, staying motivated, and adapting your activities as you age.

What to Expect

In the following chapters, we will break down the process of becoming and staying active into manageable steps:

1. ***Understanding the Risks of a Sedentary Lifestyle***: We'll explore how a lack of physical activity impacts your health and why it's crucial to get moving.

2. ***The Benefits of Physical Activity***: Discover the extensive benefits that regular exercise can bring to your body and mind.

3. ***Creating an Active Lifestyle Plan***: Learn how to set realistic goals, choose activities you enjoy, and build a sustainable routine.

4. ***Getting Started with Physical Activity***: Find out how to select the right exercises and create a balanced workout plan that fits your life.

5. ***Overcoming Common Barriers to Physical Activity***: Identify and address the obstacles that might be holding you back.

6. ***Staying Active as You Age***: Adapt your fitness routine to suit the changes in your body as you grow older.

7. ***Building a Long-Term Active Lifestyle***: Embrace a holistic approach to wellness that includes regular physical activity, nutrition, and mental health.

A Journey of Transformation

Embarking on this journey requires patience and persistence, but the rewards are immense. By taking small, consistent steps, you can transform your health and well-being. Remember, it's not about perfection but progress. Each step you take is a victory in itself.

We hope this book inspires you to embrace a more active lifestyle and provides you with the tools and confidence to make lasting changes. So let's get started on this exciting journey to becoming more active at any age. Your future self will thank you.

Section 1:
Understanding Sedentary Lifestyle

What is a Sedentary Lifestyle?

A sedentary lifestyle is characterized by a significant amount of sitting or lying down with very little to no physical activity. This lifestyle has become increasingly prevalent in modern society due to advances in technology and changes in work and leisure habits. From office jobs that require long hours in front of a computer to the ease of streaming entertainment, the opportunities for physical inactivity are abundant.

Engaging in a sedentary lifestyle means spending more than half of your waking hours in low-energy activities such as sitting, reclining, or lying down. This lack of movement can lead to a variety of health issues that affect both physical and mental well-being.

Health Risks Associated with Sedentary Behavior

While sitting in itself isn't harmful, prolonged periods of inactivity can lead to severe health consequences. Here are some of the primary health risks associated with a sedentary lifestyle:

1. Cardiovascular Diseases

→ Increased Risk of Heart Disease: Lack of physical activity can lead to poor cardiovascular health, raising the risk of heart attacks and strokes.

→ Hypertension: Sedentary behavior contributes to high blood pressure, a significant risk factor for cardiovascular diseases.

2. Obesity

→ Weight Gain: Prolonged inactivity slows down metabolism, leading to weight gain and obesity, which are risk factors for several other diseases.

→ Metabolic Syndrome: A cluster of conditions including increased blood pressure, high blood sugar, excess body fat around the waist, and abnormal cholesterol levels.

3. Type 2 Diabetes

→ Insulin Resistance: Inactivity can lead to the body becoming resistant to insulin, a hormone that regulates blood sugar, increasing the risk of developing type 2 diabetes.

4. Musculoskeletal Problems

→ Weak Muscles and Bones: Lack of exercise can cause muscle atrophy and weakened bones, making you more susceptible to injuries.

→ Joint Problems: Sedentary lifestyles can lead to stiffness and pain in the joints, contributing to conditions such as arthritis.

5. Mental Health Issues

➜ Increased Stress and Anxiety: Physical inactivity can contribute to higher levels of stress and anxiety, affecting overall mental health.

➜ Depression: Regular exercise is known to boost mood and alleviate symptoms of depression, whereas inactivity can have the opposite effect.

6. Reduced Lifespan

➜ Higher Mortality Rates: Studies have shown that sedentary lifestyles are associated with a higher risk of early death from various causes, including heart disease and cancer.

Common Causes and Patterns of Sedentary Living

Several factors contribute to a sedentary lifestyle. Understanding these can help you identify and mitigate them in your own life.

1. **Work Environment**

➜ Desk Jobs: Many people spend their workdays seated at a desk, leading to prolonged periods of inactivity.

➜ Remote Work: The increase in remote work due to technology and global events has made it easier to remain sedentary at home.

2. **Technology**

➜ Entertainment: The convenience of streaming services, video games, and social media keeps people glued to screens for hours on end.

➜ Communication: Advances in communication technology reduce the need for physical movement. Why walk to a colleague's desk when you can send an email or a message?

3. **Transportation**

➜ Car Dependency: Many urban and suburban areas are designed in ways that prioritize car travel over walking or cycling.

→ Public Transport: Commuting by bus or train often involves long periods of sitting.

4. **Leisure Activities**

→ Sedentary Hobbies: Reading, watching TV, and other hobbies that involve sitting for extended periods are popular and contribute to a lack of physical activity.

→ Convenience of Services: Home delivery services for food and groceries reduce the need to walk or drive to stores.

Real-Life Example: The Desk Job Trap

Consider John, a 45-year-old software developer. He spends about 8-10 hours a day sitting at his desk. After work, he unwinds by watching TV or playing video games. On weekends, he drives to nearby places instead of walking. Over time, John noticed he was gaining weight, felt more stressed, and had frequent back pain.

This pattern is common and highlights the subtle yet significant impact of a sedentary lifestyle.

Making the Change: A Call to Action

Recognizing the prevalence and dangers of a sedentary lifestyle is the first step toward change. Understanding these risks can motivate you to integrate more physical activity into your daily routine. Small changes, such as standing while working, taking short walks during breaks, and choosing active leisure activities, can significantly improve your health and well-being.

This detailed and engaging section can set the tone for the rest of the ebook, providing readers with a solid understanding of the sedentary lifestyle and the motivation to overcome it. Next, you can build on this foundation by developing the subsequent sections with similar depth and engagement.

Section 2:

Benefits of Staying Active

Physical Health Benefits

Cardiovascular Health

Engaging in regular physical activity significantly improves cardiovascular health. When you exercise, your heart rate increases, improving blood flow and strengthening the heart muscle. This leads to lower blood pressure, better cholesterol levels, and a reduced risk of heart disease, heart attacks, and strokes.

Real-Life Example:

Maria, a 60-year-old retired teacher, started a daily walking routine on her doctor's advice. Over six months, she noticed a significant drop in her blood pressure, increased energy levels, and an overall feeling of well-being.

Engaging Tip:

Incorporate 30 minutes of moderate-intensity aerobic exercise into your daily routine, such as brisk walking, swimming, or cycling.

Muscle Strength and Flexibility

Strength training exercises like weight lifting, resistance band workouts, and bodyweight exercises build muscle mass and improve bone density. This is crucial for preventing osteoporosis and reducing the risk of fractures as you age. Flexibility exercises, such as yoga and stretching, enhance joint mobility and reduce the risk of injuries, allowing for better balance and coordination in daily activities.

Engaging Tip:

Try a simple routine:

→ *Strength: 3 sets of 10-15 repetitions of squats, push-ups, and lunges.*

→ *Flexibility: Spend 10 minutes daily on stretching exercises that focus on major muscle groups.*

Real-Life Example:

James, a 50-year-old office worker, started incorporating strength training into his weekly routine. After three months, he noticed improved muscle tone, better posture, and fewer backaches.

Mental Health Benefits

Reduced Stress and Anxiety

Physical activity stimulates the production of endorphins, the body's natural mood elevators. Regular exercise reduces levels of the body's stress hormones, such as adrenaline and cortisol, leading to a more relaxed state of mind. Activities like running, cycling, or even brisk walking can help clear your mind and provide a sense of calm.

Real-Life Example:

David, a 35-year-old engineer, found that jogging in the park after work significantly reduced his stress levels. He felt more relaxed and better able to handle work pressures.

Engaging Tip:

Incorporate activities you enjoy into your routine to keep stress at bay. This could be anything from dancing to gardening.

Improved Mood and Cognitive Function

Exercise has been shown to alleviate symptoms of depression and anxiety. Activities like aerobic exercise and resistance training have positive effects on mood. Furthermore, physical activity enhances brain function, improving memory, learning, and overall cognitive performance.

Engaging Fact:

Studies show that people who exercise regularly have a 30% lower risk of depression and a 20% lower risk of developing Alzheimer's disease.

Real-Life Example:

Sarah, a 40-year-old graphic designer, started a morning yoga routine. She found that it not only improved her flexibility but also boosted her mood and concentration throughout the day.

Social and Emotional Benefits

Engaging in physical activities often involves social interaction, which can enhance your sense of community and emotional well-being. Whether it's joining a local sports team, a dance class, or simply walking with a friend, these social connections provide support, motivation, and a sense of belonging.

Real-Life Example:

Linda joined a local yoga class, where she not only improved her flexibility and strength but also made new friends. The sense of community kept her motivated and engaged in regular exercise.

Engaging Tip:

Look for local groups or clubs that match your interests. Whether it's a running group, a hiking club, or a dance class, social interactions can make physical activity more enjoyable and sustainable.

Staying active is essential for overall health and well-being, offering a range of physical, mental, and social benefits. By incorporating regular physical activity into your life, you can reduce the risk of numerous health issues, enhance your mood and cognitive functions, and build a supportive social network. Start small, stay consistent, and choose activities you enjoy to create a sustainable and enjoyable active lifestyle.

Section 3:

Assessing Your Current Activity Level

Self-Assessment Tools and Techniques

Understanding your current activity level is the first step toward making meaningful changes. Self-assessment tools and techniques help you identify how much you move each day and where you can improve.

Activity Trackers

Modern technology offers a range of activity trackers that can monitor your daily movements, such as:

→ Fitbit

→ Apple Watch

→ Smartphone Apps: Apps like MyFitnessPal and Google Fit track steps, active minutes, and calories burned.

These devices and apps provide valuable insights into your activity patterns, helping you set and achieve your fitness goals.

Engaging Tip:

Set a daily step goal, such as 10,000 steps, and use your tracker to monitor your progress. Celebrate small milestones to stay motivated.

Activity Log

Keeping an activity log is a simple yet effective way to track your daily activities. Note the duration and type of activities, such as sitting, walking, exercising, and sleeping. Reviewing your log helps identify patterns and areas for improvement.

Sample Activity Log:

Time of Day	Activity	Duration
7:00 AM	Walking	30 minutes

8:00 AM	Sitting (Work)	2 hours
10:00 AM	Stretch Break	10 minutes
12:00 PM	Lunch (Sitting)	1 hour
1:00 PM	Sitting (Work)	3 hours
4:00 PM	Walking Break	15 minutes
5:00 PM	Sitting (Commute)	30 minutes
6:00 PM	Dinner (Sitting)	1 hour
7:00 PM	Yoga	20 minutes
8:00 PM	Watching TV	2 hours
10:00 PM	Sleeping	8 hours

Engaging Tip:

Use colorful markers or stickers to highlight periods of activity and inactivity in your log. This visual representation can motivate you to move more.

Online Questionnaires

Online questionnaires, such as the International Physical Activity Questionnaire (IPAQ), provide a structured way to assess your physical activity levels. These questionnaires consider various aspects of your daily routine, including work, transportation, and leisure activities.

Engaging Tip:

Complete the IPAQ and set a reminder to retake it every few months to track your progress and adjust your goals as needed.

Understanding Your Baseline

Once you've gathered data from your activity tracker, log, or questionnaire, you can analyze your baseline activity level. This baseline helps you understand your starting point and set realistic goals.

Key Metrics to Consider:

➔ Daily Steps: Aim for a minimum of 7,500 steps per day.

➔ Active Minutes: Strive for at least 150 minutes of moderate-intensity or 75 minutes of vigorous-intensity activity per week.

➔ Sitting Time: Try to limit prolonged sitting periods and incorporate movement breaks.

Real-Life Example:

Jane, a 45-year-old accountant, used an activity tracker and log for a week. She discovered she was only taking about 3,000 steps per day and sitting for long periods without breaks. This insight motivated her to make small changes, like taking short walks during breaks and standing while working.

Setting Realistic and Achievable Goals

Setting goals is crucial for maintaining motivation and tracking progress. When setting your goals, ensure they are SMART: Specific, Measurable, Achievable, Relevant, and Time-bound.

SMART Goal Example:

➔ Specific: "*I want to increase my daily step count.*"

➔ Measurable: "*I will aim for 7,500 steps per day.*"

➔ Achievable: "*I will start by adding a 15-minute walk to my lunch break.*"

➔ Relevant: "*Increasing my steps will improve my overall fitness and energy levels.*"

➔ Time-bound: "*I will achieve this goal within the next month.*"

Engaging Tip:

Write down your goals and place them where you can see them daily, such as on your fridge or as a screensaver on your phone.

Real-Life Example:

Mark, a 50-year-old teacher, set a goal to reduce his sitting time by incorporating standing meetings and walking during phone calls. Over three months, he noticed a decrease in back pain and an increase in his overall energy levels.

Assessing your current activity level is a crucial step in overcoming a sedentary lifestyle. By using activity trackers, keeping an activity log, and completing online questionnaires, you can gain a clear understanding of your baseline activity. Setting SMART goals helps you stay motivated and make measurable progress. Remember, the journey to an active lifestyle begins with small, consistent steps.

Section 4:
Getting Started with Physical Activity

Choosing the Right Activities

Starting a new exercise routine can be daunting, especially if you're not sure where to begin. The key is to choose activities that you enjoy and that fit your current fitness level. Here are some types of exercises to consider:

Low-Impact Exercises

Low-impact exercises are gentle on the joints, making them suitable for beginners and those with physical limitations. These activities can help you build a strong fitness foundation without overexerting yourself.

Examples:

- → Walking: An easy way to start, requiring no special equipment.

- → Swimming: Provides a full-body workout and is great for joint health.

- → Cycling: Whether stationary or on the road, it's an excellent cardiovascular workout.

Engaging Tip:

Find scenic routes or local parks to make your walks more enjoyable. Consider joining a walking group for social interaction and motivation.

Strength Training

Building muscle strength is essential for overall health and can be achieved through various methods. Strength training not only improves muscle mass but also enhances bone density and metabolism.

Examples:

→ Bodyweight Exercises: Push-ups, squats, and lunges can be done anywhere and don't require equipment.

→ Resistance Bands: Portable and versatile, perfect for home workouts.

→ Free Weights: Dumbbells and kettlebells offer a wide range of exercises.

Engaging Tip:

Start with light weights and gradually increase as you become more comfortable. Ensure proper form to prevent injury, and consider working with a personal trainer initially.

Flexibility and Balance Exercises

Flexibility and balance are crucial for preventing injuries and maintaining overall mobility, especially as you age. These exercises can be easily integrated into your daily routine.

Examples:

➜ Yoga: Improves flexibility, strength, and mental clarity.

➜ Tai Chi: A gentle practice that enhances balance and reduces stress.

➜ Stretching: Simple stretches targeting major muscle groups.

Engaging Tip:

Join a local yoga or Tai Chi class to learn proper techniques and enjoy the social benefits of group exercise.

Creating a Routine

Establishing a consistent routine is vital for making physical activity a regular part of your life. Start small and build up gradually to avoid burnout and injury.

Starting Small and Building Up

Begin with manageable goals and gradually increase the intensity and duration of your workouts. This approach helps your body adapt and reduces the risk of injury.

Engaging Tip:

Set a weekly schedule with specific times for your workouts. Treat these appointments as non-negotiable, just like any other important commitment.

Sample Beginner Routine:

➔ Monday: 15-minute walk

➔ Tuesday: 20 minutes of strength training with resistance bands

➔ Wednesday: 10-minute stretching routine

➔ Thursday: 15-minute walk

➔ Friday: 20 minutes of yoga

➔ Saturday: 30-minute swim

➔ Sunday: Rest day or gentle stretching

Incorporating Activity into Daily Life

Look for opportunities to add movement throughout your day. Small changes can accumulate and have a significant impact on your overall activity level.

Examples:

➜ Take the stairs: Skip the elevator whenever possible.

➜ Walk or bike for errands: Combine exercise with daily tasks.

➜ Desk stretches: Incorporate short stretching breaks if you have a desk job.

➜ Active breaks: Use TV commercials or work breaks to do a few exercises.

Engaging Tip:

Set reminders on your phone to prompt you to move every hour. Even a few minutes of activity can make a difference.

Staying Motivated

Motivation is key to maintaining a long-term exercise routine. Here are some strategies to keep you inspired and committed.

Tracking Progress

Monitoring your progress helps you see improvements and stay motivated. Use tools like activity trackers, fitness apps, or a simple journal to record your workouts.

Engaging Tip:

Celebrate milestones, such as reaching a new personal best or sticking to your routine for a month. Reward yourself with something enjoyable, like a new workout outfit or a relaxing massage.

Finding a Support System

Having a support system can make a significant difference in maintaining your motivation. Friends, family, or workout groups can provide encouragement and accountability.

Examples:

➜ Workout Buddy: Partner with a friend or family member to exercise together.

➜ Join a Class: Fitness classes offer structured workouts and a sense of community.

➜ Online Communities: Connect with others on social media or fitness forums.

Engaging Tip:

Share your fitness goals and achievements with your support system. Their encouragement can boost your motivation and keep you accountable.

Real-Life Example:

Tom, a 55-year-old accountant, struggled to stay active on his own. He joined a local running club and found the camaraderie and support incredibly motivating. He not only improved his fitness but also made new friends.

Starting an exercise routine doesn't have to be overwhelming. By choosing activities you enjoy, creating a manageable routine, and finding ways to stay motivated, you can make physical activity a regular and enjoyable part of your life. Remember, the key is to start small, build up gradually, and find a support system that encourages you along the way.

Section 5:
Overcoming Common Barriers to Physical Activity

Identifying and Addressing Common Barriers

Starting and maintaining a physical activity routine can be challenging. Understanding and addressing common barriers can help you stay on track.

Lack of Time

One of the most common barriers is the perception of not having enough time to exercise. Busy schedules can make it difficult to find time for physical activity.

Strategies to Overcome:

→ Prioritize Exercise: Treat it as an essential part of your day, just like eating or sleeping.

→ Break It Down: Divide your exercise into shorter, manageable sessions throughout the day. For example, three 10-minute walks can be as effective as one 30-minute session.

→ Incorporate Activity into Routine Tasks: Walk or bike to work, do household chores vigorously, or take active breaks during the day.

Real-Life Example:

Anna, a 40-year-old lawyer, struggled to find time for exercise. She started doing short, high-intensity workouts during her lunch breaks and found it easier to stay consistent.

Lack of Motivation

Staying motivated can be difficult, especially when starting a new routine. Finding ways to keep your enthusiasm high is crucial for long-term success.

Strategies to Overcome:

→ Set Clear Goals: Having specific, measurable goals can keep you focused and motivated.

→ Find Enjoyable Activities: Choose exercises that you find fun and engaging.

→ Reward Yourself: Celebrate milestones with non-food rewards, like a new book, a movie night, or a spa day.

Real-Life Example:

Brian, a 35-year-old teacher, lacked motivation to exercise. He discovered that joining a local basketball league made workouts enjoyable and gave him something to look forward to each week.

Physical Limitations and Health Issues

Physical limitations or chronic health issues can make it difficult to engage in certain types of physical activity. However, with the right approach, you can still stay active.

Strategies to Overcome:

→ Consult a Professional: Speak with a doctor or physical therapist to design a safe and effective exercise plan tailored to your needs.

→ Adapt Activities: Modify exercises to fit your abilities. For example, chair exercises can be a good option for those with mobility issues.

→ Start Slow: Begin with low-impact activities and gradually increase intensity as you become more comfortable.

Real-Life Example:

Linda, a 60-year-old with arthritis, found it difficult to do high-impact exercises. Her physical therapist recommended water aerobics, which provided a low-impact, full-body workout that alleviate joint pain.

Lack of Access to Facilities or Equipment

Not having access to a gym or exercise equipment can feel like a significant barrier, but there are many ways to stay active without them.

Strategies to Overcome:

➔ Bodyweight Exercises: Many effective exercises, like squats, lunges, and push-ups, require no equipment.

➔ Use Household Items: Cans of food or water bottles can serve as makeshift weights.

➔ Outdoor Activities: Walking, running, hiking, and cycling are great options that don't require a gym.

Real-Life Example:

Tom, a 30-year-old student, couldn't afford a gym membership. He started using free online workout videos and found creative ways to stay active at home using everyday items.

Boredom

Doing the same routine can become monotonous, leading to boredom and decreased motivation.

Strategies to Overcome:

→ Variety: Mix up your routine by trying different activities, such as dancing, hiking, or playing a sport.

→ Change of Scenery: Exercise in different locations, like parks, trails, or different neighborhoods.

→ Join Classes: Group classes can offer a fun and social way to stay active.

Real-Life Example:

Emily, a 28-year-old marketer, felt bored with her treadmill workouts. She started taking dance classes and discovered a new passion that kept her excited about staying active.

Creating a Supportive Environment

Your environment plays a significant role in your ability to maintain a physical activity routine. Creating a supportive environment can help you overcome barriers and stay consistent.

Home Environment

Make your home conducive to physical activity by designating a space for exercise and keeping your workout gear accessible.

Strategies:

- ➜ Create a Workout Space: Dedicate a small area of your home for exercising.
- ➜ Keep Equipment Handy: Store your exercise mat, weights, and other gear where you can easily access them.
- ➜ Visual Reminders: Use sticky notes or a whiteboard to remind yourself of your fitness goals and daily activities.

Engaging Tip:

Personalize your workout space with motivational quotes, photos, or music that inspires you.

Social Support

Having a support network can greatly enhance your motivation and commitment to staying active.

Strategies:

→ Workout Buddy: Find a friend or family member to exercise with.

→ Join Groups: Participate in local fitness groups or online communities.

→ Share Goals: Tell your friends and family about your fitness goals so they can encourage and support you.

Real-Life Example:

Jack, a 50-year-old salesman, struggled to stay motivated alone. He joined a local hiking club and found the social interaction and group accountability incredibly motivating.

Staying Flexible and Adjusting Your Plan

Life can be unpredictable, and it's essential to remain flexible and willing to adjust your fitness plan as needed.

Strategies:

→ Adapt to Changes: If your schedule changes, find new times for your workouts.

→ Be Kind to Yourself: It's okay to miss a workout occasionally. Focus on getting back on track rather than dwelling on missed sessions.

→ Reevaluate Goals: Regularly assess your goals and progress, and make adjustments to keep your routine effective and engaging.

Real-Life Example:

Samantha, a 32-year-old nurse, had a fluctuating work schedule. She created a flexible workout plan that allowed her to fit in exercise during different times of the day, depending on her shifts.

Overcoming barriers to physical activity is essential for maintaining a healthy and active lifestyle. By identifying common challenges and implementing strategies to address them, you can stay committed to your fitness goals. Remember, the key is to stay flexible, seek support, and find activities that you enjoy. With the right mindset and approach, you can overcome obstacles and lead a more active, fulfilling life.

Section 6:
Staying Active as You Age

Understanding the Aging Body

As we age, our bodies undergo various changes that can impact our physical abilities and overall health. Understanding these changes can help you adapt your exercise routine to stay active and healthy.

Physical Changes

➤ Muscle Mass and Strength: After the age of 30, muscle mass and strength gradually decline, a process known as sarcopenia. Regular strength training can help slow this decline and maintain muscle function.

➤ Bone Density: Bone density decreases with age, increasing the risk of osteoporosis and fractures. Weight-bearing exercises like walking and strength training can improve bone health.

➢ Joint Health: Joints may become stiffer and less flexible over time. Low-impact exercises and flexibility training can help maintain joint health and reduce pain.

➢ Cardiovascular Health: The efficiency of the heart and lungs may decrease with age. Aerobic exercises can help maintain cardiovascular health and improve endurance.

➢ Metabolism: Metabolism tends to slow down with age, making it easier to gain weight. Regular physical activity can help manage weight and boost metabolic rate.

Real-Life Example:

Helen, a 65-year-old retired nurse, incorporated a mix of strength training, walking, and yoga into her routine. She found that her energy levels improved, and she experienced fewer aches and pains.

Tailoring Your Routine for Aging

Adapting your exercise routine to suit your aging body is crucial for staying active and preventing injuries.

Low-Impact Aerobic Exercises

Low-impact aerobic exercises are easier on the joints and provide cardiovascular benefits without excessive strain.

Examples:

- ➔ Walking: A simple and effective way to maintain cardiovascular health.
- ➔ Swimming: Offers a full-body workout and reduces joint stress.
- ➔ Cycling: Stationary or outdoor cycling provides a good cardiovascular workout.

Engaging Tip:

Join a walking group or participate in community pool classes to make these activities more social and enjoyable.

Strength Training

Strength training is essential for maintaining muscle mass and bone density as you age. Focus on exercises that work all major muscle groups.

Examples:

→ Bodyweight Exercises: Squats, push-ups, and lunges.

→ Resistance Bands: Portable and versatile for home workouts.

→ Free Weights: Dumbbells and kettlebells.

Engaging Tip:

Work with a personal trainer who specializes in older adults to ensure proper form and safety.

Flexibility and Balance Exercises

Flexibility and balance exercises help prevent falls and improve overall mobility.

Examples:

→ Yoga: Enhances flexibility, strength, and mental clarity.

→ Tai Chi: Improves balance and reduces stress.

→ Stretching: Daily stretching routine targeting major muscle groups.

Engaging Tip:

Look for local or online classes that focus on senior fitness to ensure the exercises are age-appropriate.

Real-Life Example:

George, a 70-year-old retiree, started practicing Tai Chi twice a week. He noticed significant improvements in his balance and reduced joint stiffness.

Staying Motivated and Engaged

Maintaining motivation is key to staying active as you age. Here are some strategies to keep you engaged:

Setting Realistic Goals

Set achievable goals that are specific, measurable, and time-bound. Adjust your goals as needed to reflect your progress and any changes in your health.

SMART Goal Example:

→ Specific: "I want to improve my flexibility."

→ Measurable: "I will do a 15-minute stretching routine three times a week."

→ Achievable: "I will start with beginner stretches."

→ Relevant: "Improving flexibility will enhance my mobility."

→ Time-bound: "I will achieve this within two months."

Engaging Tip:

Keep a journal to track your progress and celebrate your achievements, no matter how small.

Finding a Support System

A support system can provide encouragement and accountability, making it easier to stick to your routine.

Examples:

→ Workout Buddy: Partner with a friend or family member.

→ Join Classes: Participate in local fitness classes tailored for seniors.

→ Online Communities: Engage with others through social media or fitness forums.

Real-Life Example:

Betty, a 68-year-old grandmother, joined a local senior fitness group. The camaraderie and support from the group kept her motivated and consistent with her workouts.

Engaging Tip:

Share your fitness journey with friends and family. Their support and encouragement can be incredibly motivating.

Embracing Technology

Technology can be a helpful tool in staying active and tracking your progress.

Examples:

→ Fitness Apps: Use apps like MyFitnessPal or Fitbit to monitor your activity and set goals.

→ Online Classes: Access a wide range of exercise classes from the comfort of your home.

→ Virtual Trainers: Consider virtual training sessions with a professional to ensure you're on the right track.

Engaging Tip:

Explore fitness apps and online resources that offer senior-specific workouts and health tips.

Real-Life Example:

John, a 72-year-old tech enthusiast, used a fitness tracker to monitor his steps and joined online yoga classes. The convenience and variety helped him stay active and engaged.

Staying active as you age is crucial for maintaining overall health, mobility, and quality of life. By understanding the changes that occur in your body and tailoring your exercise routine accordingly, you can enjoy the numerous benefits of physical activity. Stay motivated by setting realistic goals, finding a support system, and embracing technology. Remember, it's never too late to start and every step you take brings you closer to a healthier, more active lifestyle.

Section 7:
Building a Long-Term Active Lifestyle

The Importance of Consistency

Creating a long-term active lifestyle is about consistency and making physical activity an integral part of your daily routine. Consistent exercise can lead to sustained health benefits, increased energy levels, and improved mental well-being.

Benefits of Consistency

→ Physical Health: Regular exercise helps maintain a healthy weight, reduces the risk of chronic diseases, and strengthens the cardiovascular system.

→ Mental Health: Consistent activity can reduce stress, anxiety, and depression, while improving mood and cognitive function.

➜ Longevity: Studies have shown that regular physical activity can increase lifespan and improve the quality of life in later years.

Engaging Tip:

Think of exercise as a non-negotiable part of your day, like brushing your teeth or eating meals. Establishing this mindset helps make it a consistent habit.

Making Exercise Enjoyable

Enjoying your exercise routine is key to maintaining it long-term. Find activities that you look forward to and that fit your lifestyle.

Exploring Different Activities

Variety keeps your routine interesting and can prevent burnout. Experiment with different types of exercises to find what you enjoy most.

Examples:

- ➜ Dance Classes: Zumba, salsa, or ballroom dancing can be fun and engaging.

- ➜ Outdoor Activities: Hiking, kayaking, or nature walks provide fresh air and a change of scenery.

- ➜ Team Sports: Joining a local league or playing pick-up games with friends.

Engaging Tip:

Make a list of activities you've always wanted to try and incorporate them into your routine. This keeps things exciting and helps you discover new passions.

Combining Exercise with Social Activities

Combining physical activity with social interactions can make exercise more enjoyable and provide additional motivation.

Examples:

> → Group Workouts: Attend fitness classes with friends or family.

> → Active Outings: Plan active outings, like bike rides or beach volleyball, with your social circle.

> → Fitness Challenges: Participate in friendly fitness challenges with colleagues or neighbors.

Engaging Tip:

Organize regular fitness meet-ups with friends or join a local exercise group. The social aspect can make workouts more fun and keep you accountable.

Real-Life Example:

Karen, a 50-year-old marketing executive, joined a weekly hiking group. The combination of exercise and social interaction kept her motivated and led to lasting friendships.

Adapting to Life Changes

Life is dynamic, and your fitness routine should be flexible enough to adapt to various life changes. Whether it's a busy work period, travel, or health issues, being adaptable ensures you can stay active regardless of circumstances.

Strategies for Busy Periods

During busy times, finding ways to incorporate exercise into your daily routine is crucial.

Examples:

- → Micro Workouts: Short, intense workouts can be effective. Try 10-minute HIIT sessions or quick yoga flows.
- → Active Commuting: Walk or bike to work if possible.
- → Incorporate Movement: Use breaks at work to do simple exercises like stretching or walking.

Engaging Tip:

Schedule your workouts like any other important appointment. Even if it's just a 10-minute session, it's better than skipping it entirely.

Staying Active While Traveling

Travel can disrupt your routine, but with a little planning, you can stay active on the go.

Examples:

➜ Hotel Gyms: Many hotels have fitness centers available for guests.

➜ Bodyweight Exercises: Pack a resistance band and do bodyweight exercises in your room.

➜ Explore on Foot: Walk or bike to explore new places instead of using taxis or public transport.

Engaging Tip:

Research fitness options at your destination before you go. Look for nearby parks, gyms, or trails to keep your routine on track.

Adjusting for Health Issues

Health issues may require modifications to your exercise routine, but they don't have to stop you from staying active.

Strategies:

→ Consult a Professional: Work with a healthcare provider or physical therapist to develop a safe exercise plan.

→ Low-Impact Options: Focus on low-impact activities like swimming, walking, or cycling.

→ Listen to Your Body: Pay attention to how your body responds and adjust your intensity accordingly.

Real-Life Example:

James, a 60-year-old with knee arthritis, switched from running to swimming. This low-impact exercise allowed him to stay active without exacerbating his condition.

Tracking Progress and Staying Accountable

Monitoring your progress and staying accountable can significantly impact your long-term success. It helps you see your improvements and keeps you motivated to continue.

Using Fitness Trackers and Apps

Fitness trackers and apps can help you set goals, track progress, and stay motivated.

Popular Options:

- ➜ Fitbit
- ➜ Apple Health
- ➜ MyFitnessPal

→ Strava

Engaging Tip:

Set daily or weekly goals on your tracker or app and regularly review your progress. Celebrate milestones to keep yourself motivated.

Keeping a Fitness Journal

A fitness journal is a simple way to record your workouts, track your progress, and reflect on your journey.

What to Include:

→ Workout Details: Date, type of exercise, duration, and intensity.

→ Goals: Short-term and long-term fitness goals.

→ Progress: Notes on improvements, challenges, and achievements.

→ Reflections: How you felt during and after workouts.

Engaging Tip:

Personalize your journal with motivational quotes, photos, or stickers. Reviewing your entries can provide a sense of accomplishment and inspire you to keep going.

Real-Life Example:

Emma, a 45-year-old artist, used a fitness journal to track her workouts and reflect on her progress. The visual record of her journey kept her motivated and helped her stay consistent.

Embracing a Holistic Approach to Wellness

Building a long-term active lifestyle involves more than just physical activity. Embracing a holistic approach to wellness can enhance your overall quality of life.

Nutrition

A balanced diet provides the fuel needed for your body to perform and recover from physical activity.

Key Points:

➔ Whole Foods: Focus on whole, nutrient-dense foods like fruits, vegetables, lean proteins, and whole grains.

➔ Hydration: Stay hydrated by drinking plenty of water throughout the day.

➔ Moderation: Enjoy treats in moderation to maintain a balanced approach.

Engaging Tip:

Experiment with new healthy recipes and share meals with friends or family to make eating well enjoyable and social.

Mental Health

Mental well-being is as important as physical health. Incorporate practices that support your mental health into your routine.

Examples:

➔ Mindfulness: Practice mindfulness or meditation to reduce stress and improve focus.

→ Sleep: Aim for 7-9 hours of quality sleep per night.

→ Social Connections: Maintain strong social connections for emotional support and happiness.

Engaging Tip:

Dedicate time each day for self-care activities that you enjoy, such as reading, gardening, or spending time with loved ones.

Real-Life Example:

Linda, a 55-year-old librarian, combined her morning walks with meditation. This routine helped her start the day with a clear mind and positive outlook.

Building a long-term active lifestyle requires consistency, enjoyment, adaptability, and a holistic approach to wellness. By making physical activity a regular and enjoyable part of your life, adapting to changes, tracking your progress, and embracing overall well-being, you can achieve lasting health and happiness. Remember, the journey is personal and unique to each individual.

Stay committed, be flexible, and enjoy the process of becoming the healthiest version of yourself.

Conclusion

Congratulations on reaching the end of "Active at Any Age: A Beginner's Guide to Overcoming a Sedentary Lifestyle." By now, you've gained a comprehensive understanding of the importance of physical activity and how it can dramatically improve your life, regardless of your age or current fitness level. This journey is just beginning, and the steps you take today will pave the way for a healthier, more vibrant future.

Recap of Key Points

Let's briefly revisit the key takeaways from this book:

1. Understanding the Risks of a Sedentary Lifestyle: A sedentary lifestyle poses significant health risks, including chronic diseases and mental health challenges. Recognizing these dangers is the first step toward change.

2. The Benefits of Physical Activity: Regular exercise offers numerous benefits, from enhancing physical health and reducing disease risk to improving mental well-being and boosting energy levels.

3. Creating an Active Lifestyle Plan: Setting realistic goals, choosing enjoyable activities, and building a sustainable routine are crucial for long-term success.

4. Getting Started with Physical Activity: Selecting the right exercises and creating a balanced workout plan tailored to your needs ensures you can start safely and effectively.

5. Overcoming Common Barriers to Physical Activity: Identifying and addressing obstacles such as time constraints, lack of motivation, physical limitations, and boredom can help you stay on track.

6. Staying Active as You Age: Adapting your fitness routine to suit the changes in your body as you age ensures you can remain active and healthy throughout your life.

7. Building a Long-Term Active Lifestyle: Embracing consistency, making exercise enjoyable, adapting to life changes, tracking progress, and adopting a holistic approach to wellness are essential for sustaining an active lifestyle.

Embracing Lifelong Fitness

Creating an active lifestyle is more than just a short-term goal; it's a lifelong commitment to your health and well-being. Remember, the journey to fitness is personal and unique. It's about finding what works for you, adapting to your body's needs, and making physical activity an integral part of your daily life.

Celebrating Your Progress

Every step you take toward a more active lifestyle is an achievement. Celebrate your progress, no matter how small. Whether it's taking the stairs instead of the elevator, completing your first 5K, or simply enjoying a daily walk, each milestone is a testament to your commitment and determination.

Staying Inspired and Motivated

Staying motivated can be challenging, but surrounding yourself with support, setting new goals, and keeping your routine fresh and enjoyable can help. Remember, it's okay to have setbacks. What matters is your ability to get back on track and keep moving forward.

The Power of Community

Don't underestimate the power of community. Engage with friends, family, and local groups to stay inspired and accountable. Share your journey, seek support, and encourage others to join you. Together, we can create a culture that values and prioritizes health and activity at every age.

Looking Ahead

As you move forward, continue to educate yourself, seek new challenges, and adapt your routine as needed. Your health is your greatest asset, and investing in it through regular physical activity will yield lifelong dividends.

Thank you for taking the time to read this book and for committing to a healthier, more active lifestyle. The steps you take today will lead to a brighter, more energetic future. Keep moving, stay motivated, and enjoy the journey to becoming the best version of yourself at any age.

Here's to a lifetime of health, happiness, and vitality. You've got this!